THINGS THAT GROSS ME OUT!

VOMIT IS SO GROSS!

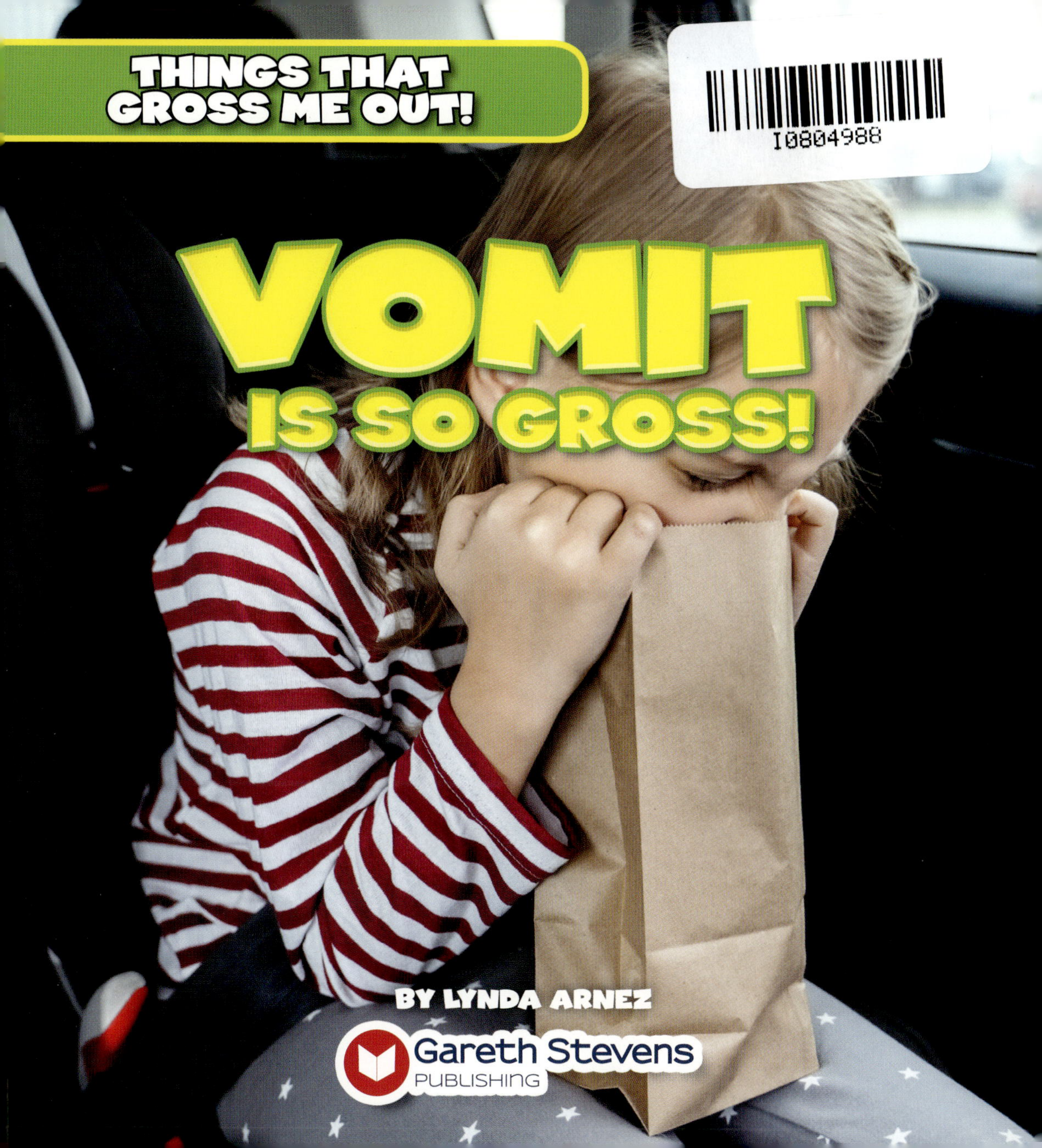

BY LYNDA ARNEZ

Gareth Stevens PUBLISHING

Please visit our website, www.garethstevens.com. For a free color catalog of all our high-quality books, call toll free 1-800-542-2595 or fax 1-877-542-2596.

Cataloging-in-Publication Data

Names: Arnéz, Lynda.
Title: Vomit is so gross! / Lynda Arnéz.
Description: Buffalo, NY : Gareth Stevens Publishing, 2026. | Series: Things that gross me out! | Includes glossary and index.
Identifiers: ISBN 9781482471502 (pbk.) | ISBN 9781482471519 (library bound) | ISBN 9781482471526 (ebook)
Subjects: LCSH: Vomiting–Juvenile literature. | Nausea–Juvenile literature. | Human physiology–Juvenile literature.
Classification: LCC RB150.N38 A76 2026 | DDC 612.3–dc23

Published in 2026 by
Gareth Stevens Publishing
2544 Clinton Street
Buffalo, NY 14224

Designer: Tanya Dellaccio Keeney
Editor: Kristen Nelson

Photo credits: Cover Ira Lichi/Shutterstock.com; p. 5 antoniodiaz/Shutterstock.com; p. 7 CGN089/Shutterstock.com; p. 9 alexandrabadashovaa/Shutterstock.com; pp. 11, 21 Prostock-studio/Shutterstock.com; p. 13 Red Stock/Shutterstock.com; p. 15 photolin/Shutterstock.com; p. 17 FotoDuets/Shutterstock.com; p. 19 Halfpoint/Shutterstock.com.

Printed in the United States of America

CPSIA compliance information: Batch #CS26GS: For further information contact Gareth Stevens at 1-800-542-2595.

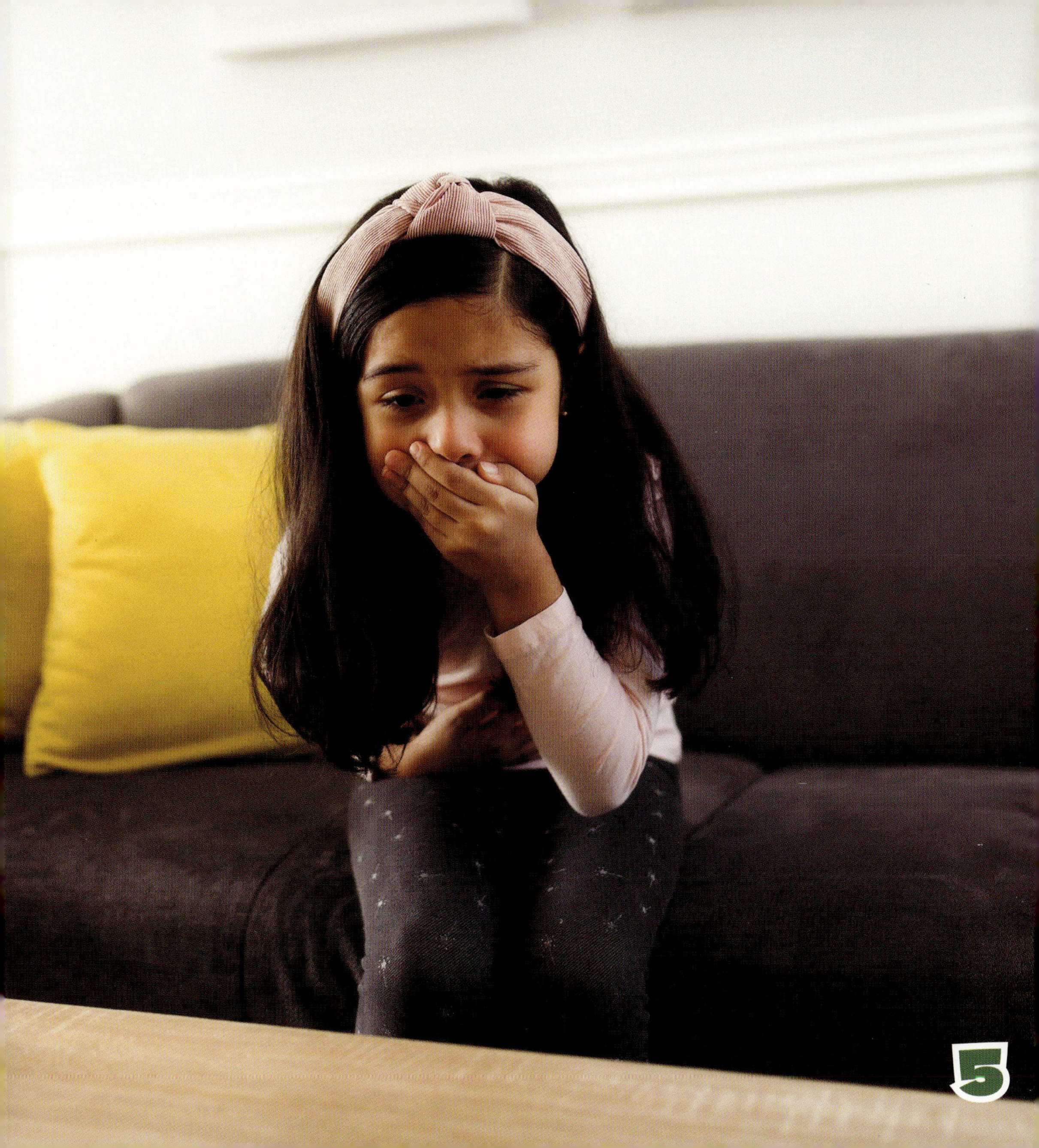

When your body pushes the contents of your **stomach** back out through your mouth, that's vomiting. What comes out is called vomit too. Vomiting is usually pretty forceful. It might hurt. And it keeps happening until the body gets rid of what it needs to!

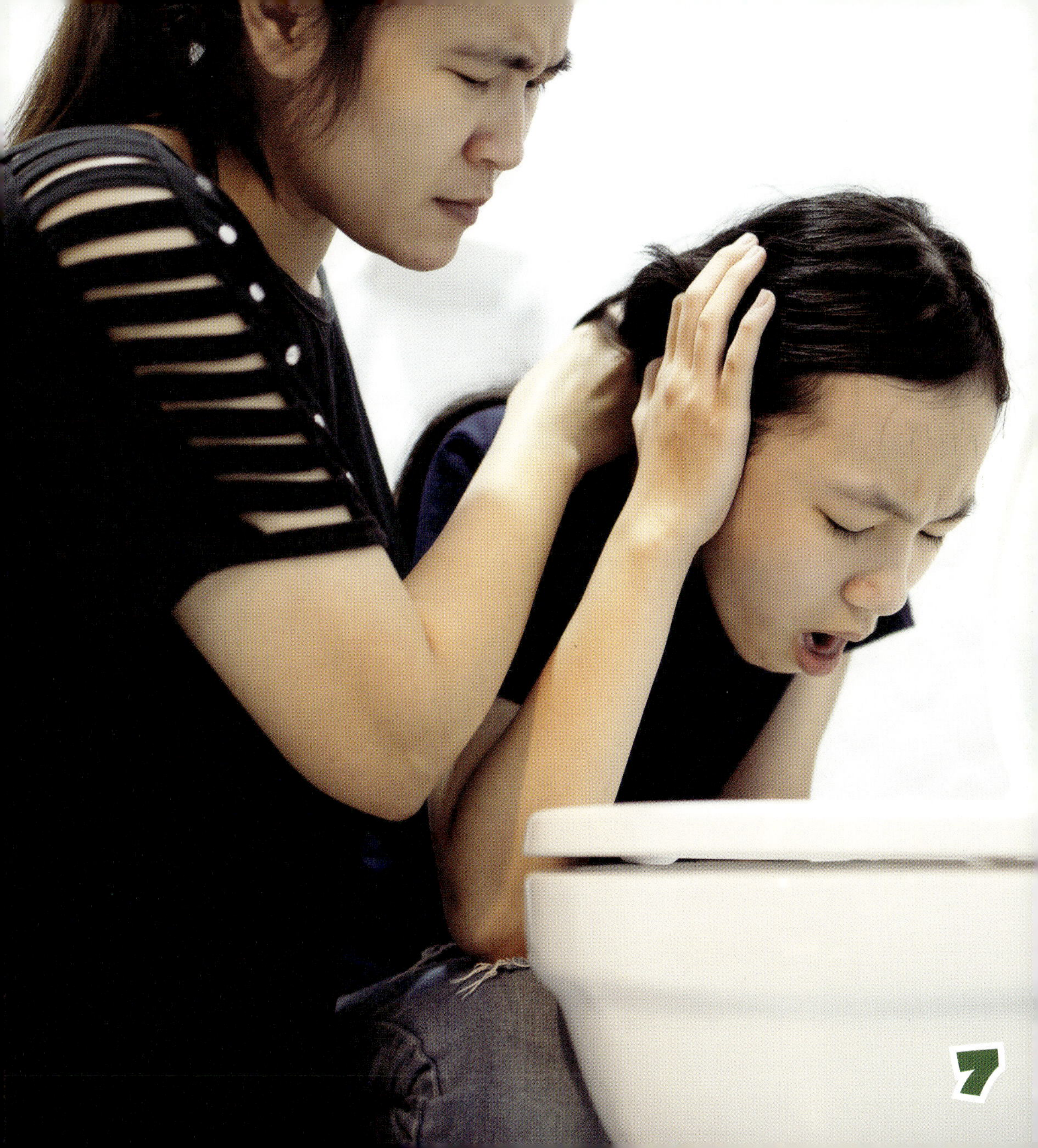

Why You Would Vomit

A kid might vomit for a lot of reasons. Most of the time, it's because of sickness. You might have an **infection** in your stomach or **intestines**. Sometimes this is called the "stomach flu." It can be caused by **bacteria** or other germs.

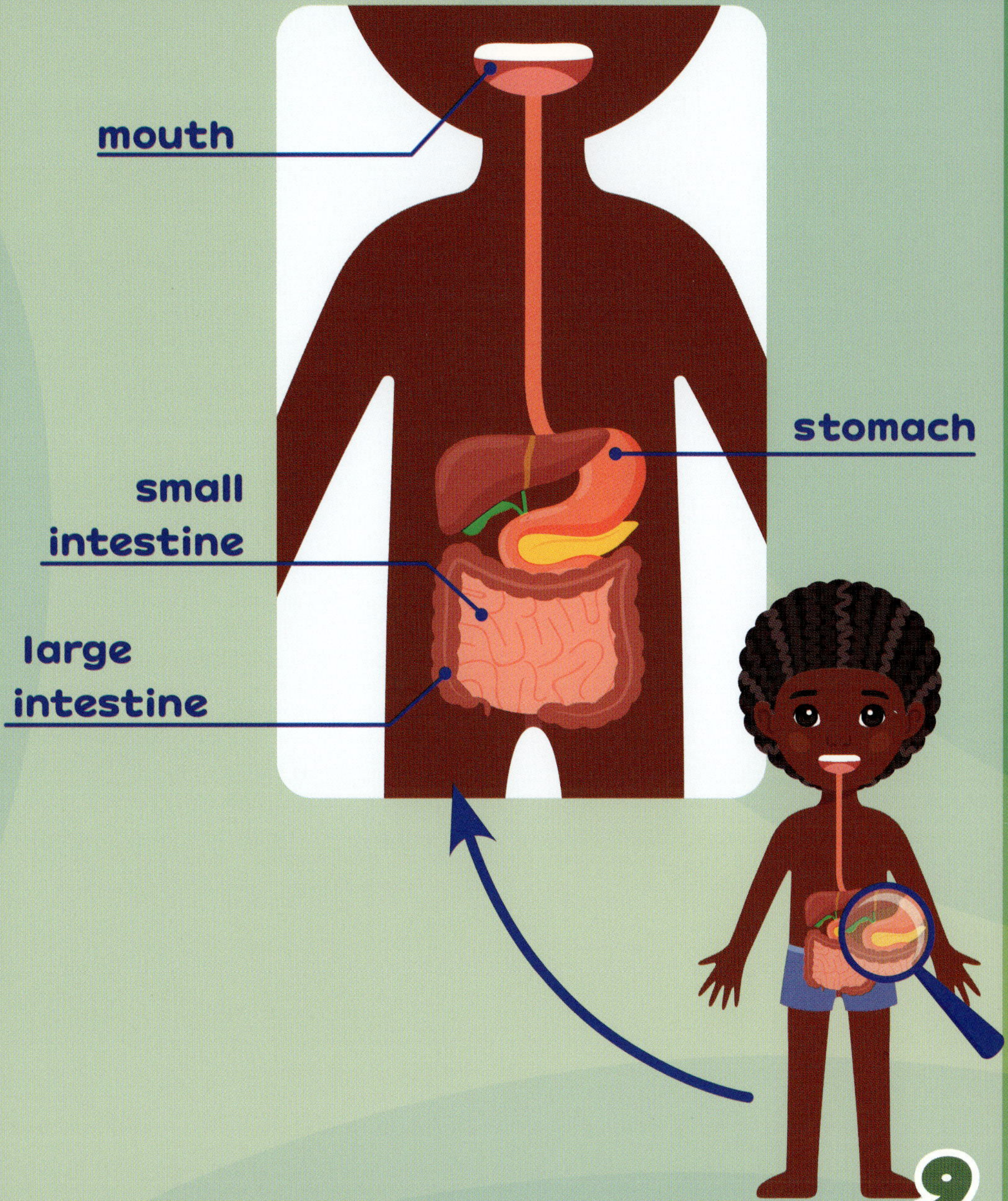
mouth
stomach
small intestine
large intestine

Eating food that has gone bad or has bad bacteria in it can make you sick too. This is called food poisoning. Some people may vomit, or have **nausea**, from driving in a car, riding on a boat, or going on a spinning ride. This is called motion sickness.

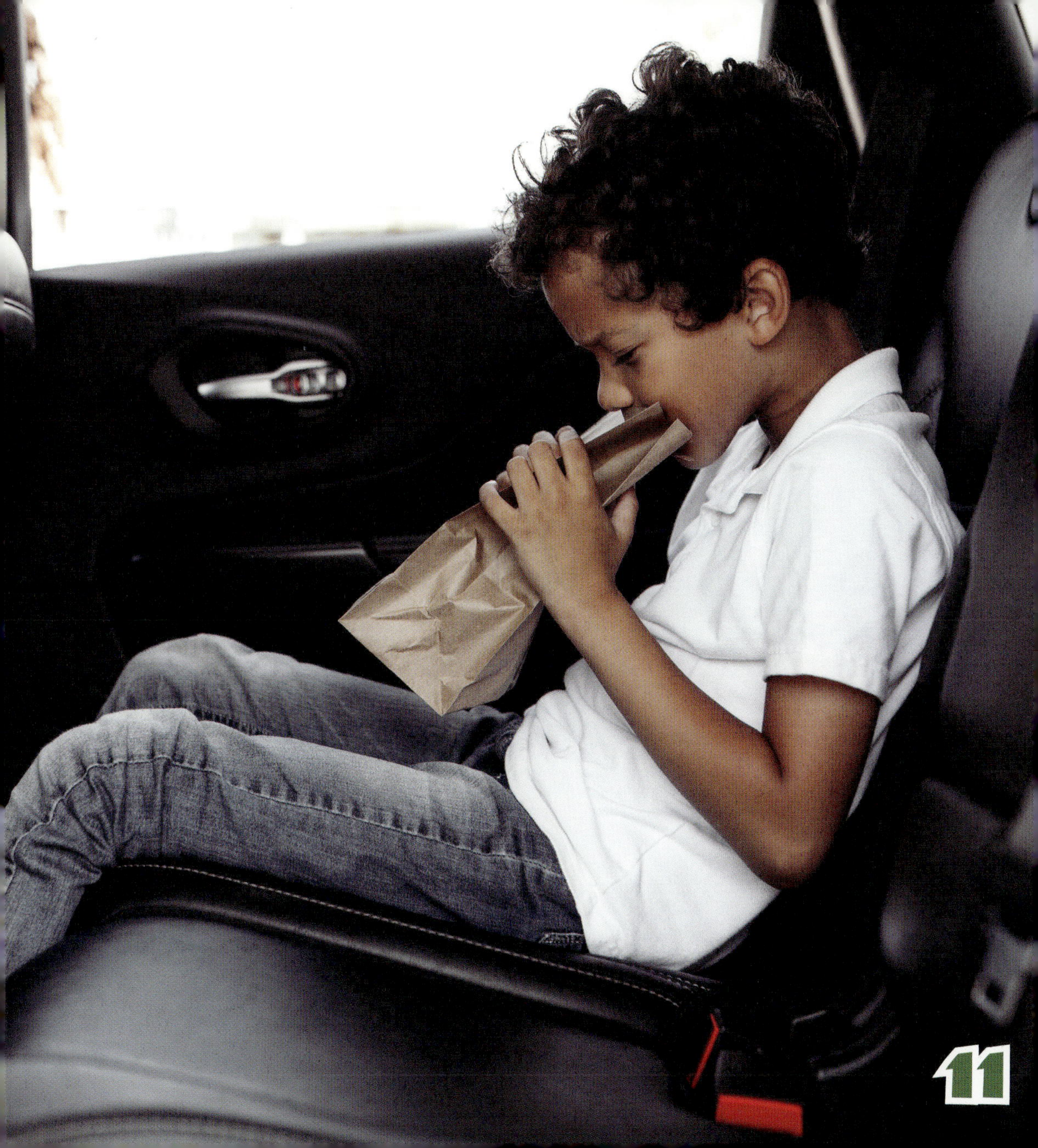

How It Happens

Chewed food moves from the mouth to the stomach, through the intestines, and out of the body as poop. But, when you are sick or eat something bad, your stomach muscles and intestines **contract**. They push the food back up to your mouth and ... YUCK!

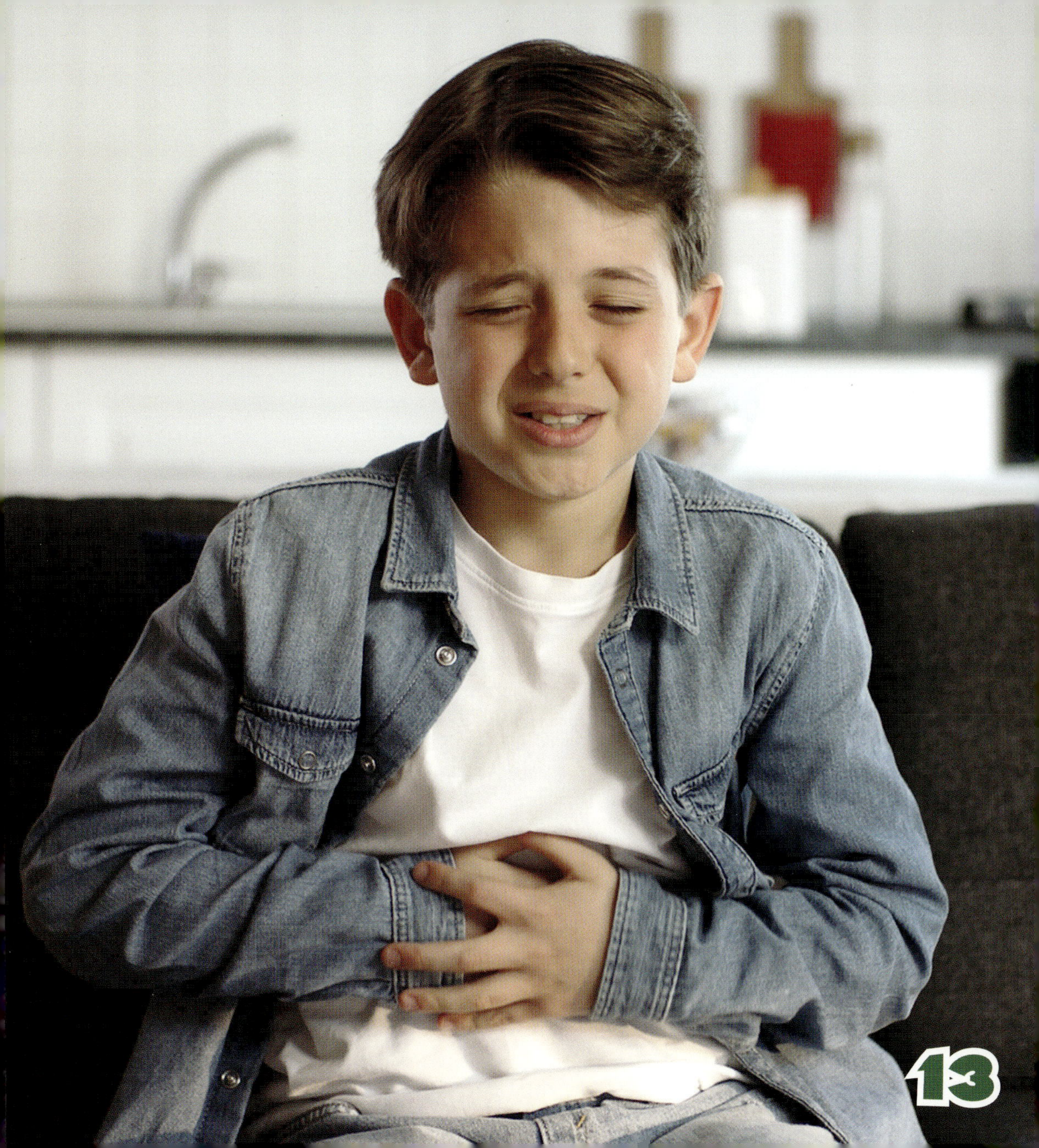

That Looks ... GROSS!

Vomit is a mix of matter. It has food that's partly **digested** in it. This may make your puke a color, such as red if you just ate some watermelon. Vomit has water and saliva, or spit, in it. It also contains stomach acid, or the matter that helps break down the food you eat.

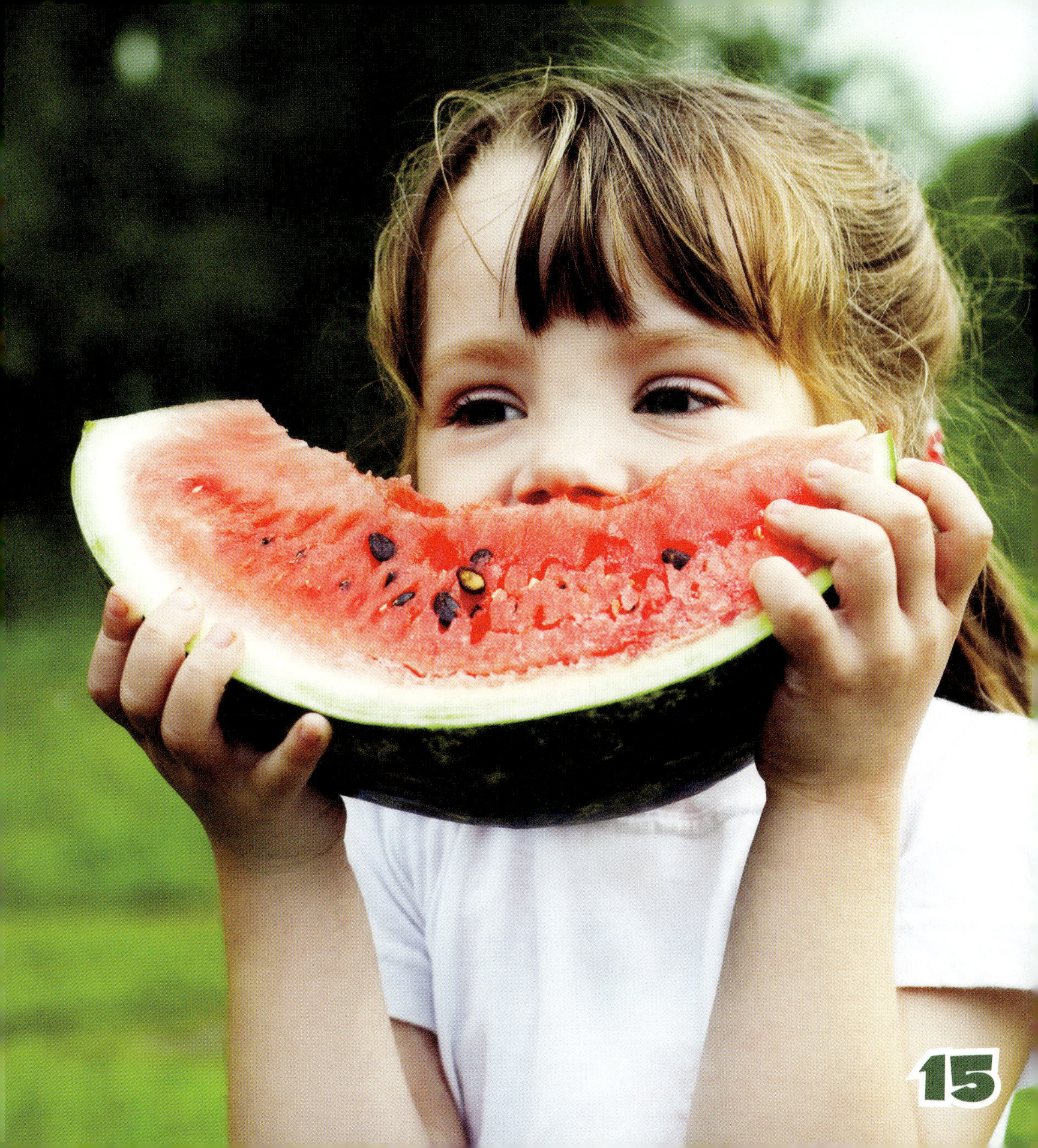

Taking Care of Yourself

Most of the time, vomiting only lasts about a day. Kids might have a **fever** or **diarrhea** during that time as well. The best thing to do is rest. You should sip water or other special drinks your parent or caregiver gives you.

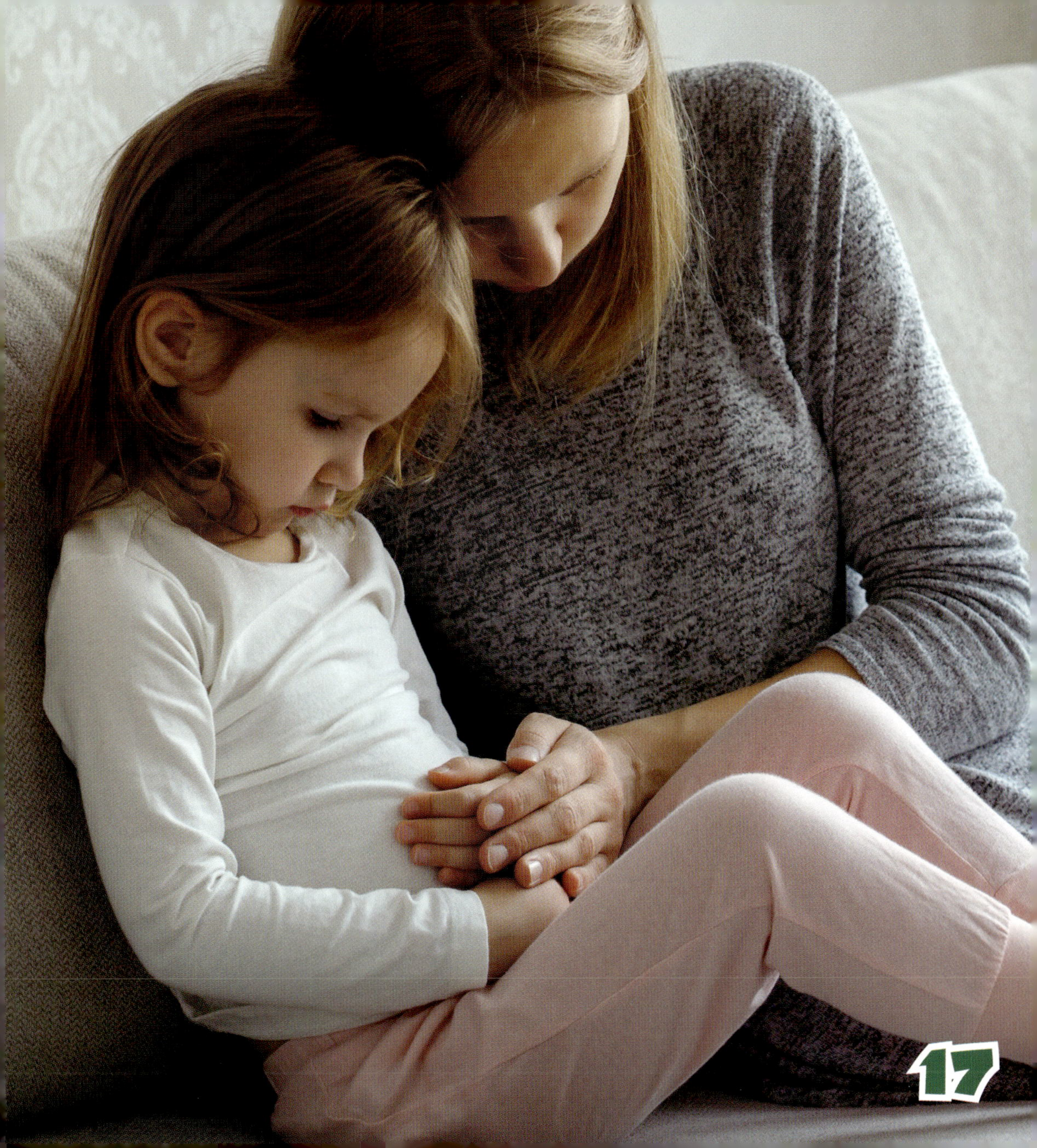

Dehydration

Sometimes, a kid might throw up so much that they can't keep any drinks down. They may become dehydrated. This means their body has lost too much water to work the way it should. They may have to go to the hospital to get the **fluids** they need.

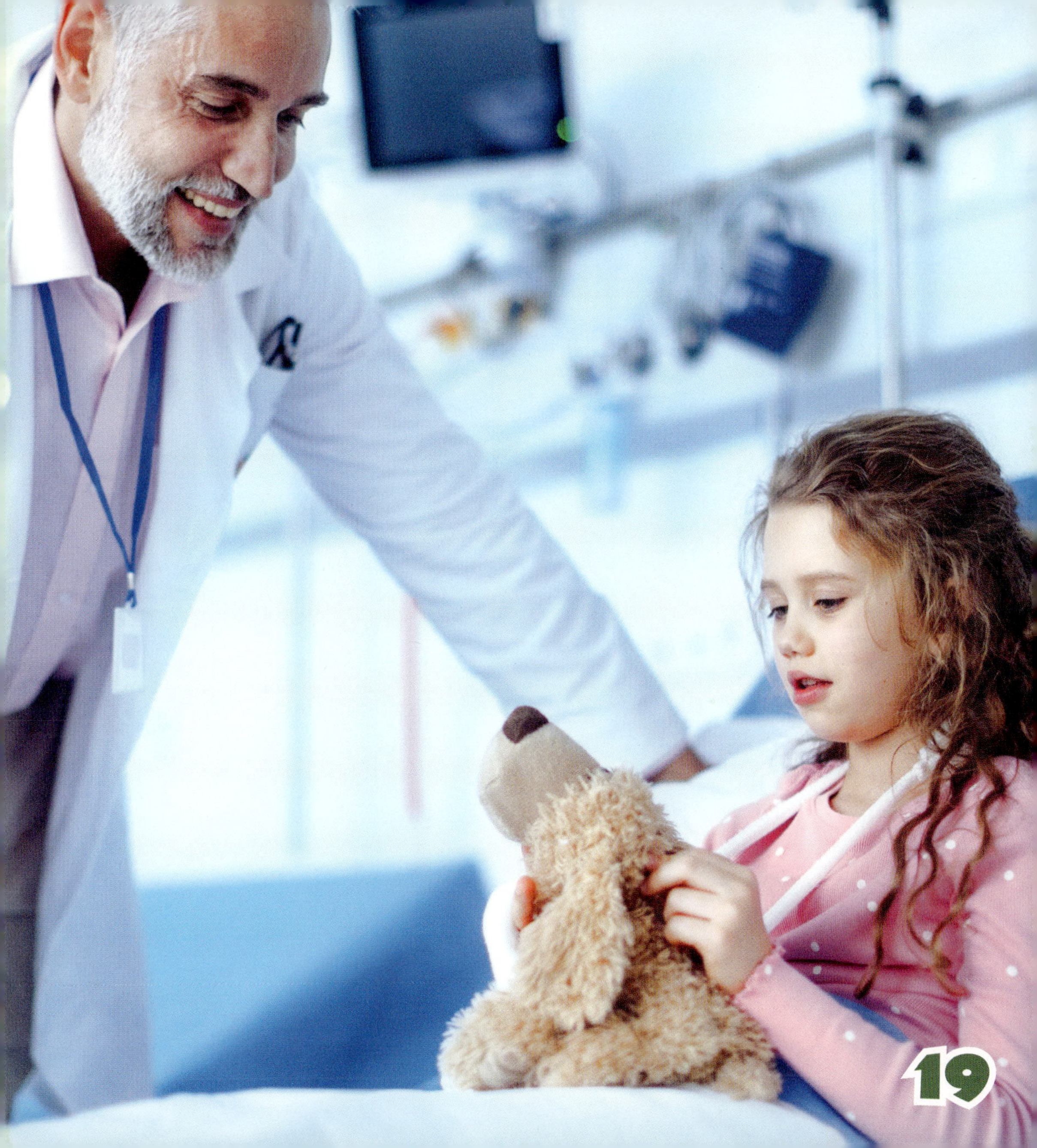

Animal Vomit

Animals throw up too. They do so for many of the same reasons people do. Even grosser, some animals eat their puke. You may have seen your pet dog do this! They may like how it tastes or are trying to clean it up, among other reasons. Ew!

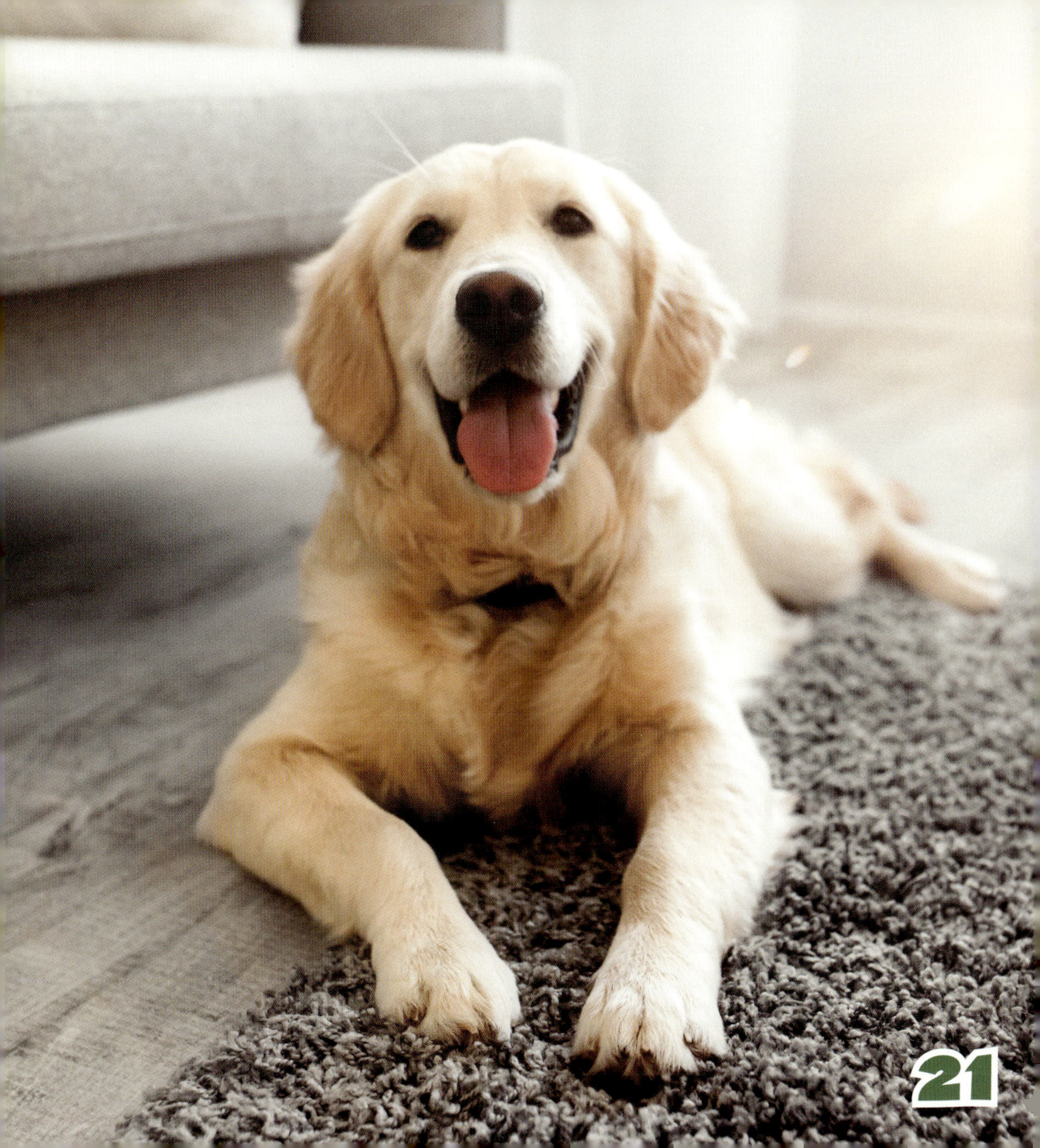

GLOSSARY

bacteria: Tiny living things that can only be seen with a microscope.

contract: Tighten.

diarrhea: A watery poop.

digest: To break down.

fever: A body temperature higher than normal or healthy.

fluid: Something that flows like a liquid.

infection: The spread of germs inside the body, causing illness.

intestine: A tube in the body that helps digest food.

nausea: A feeling in the stomach like you're going to throw up.

stomach: A part of the body where food is digested.

FOR MORE INFORMATION

BOOKS

Branzei, Sylvia. *Nitty-Gritty Grossology: Over 101 Disgusting Facts*. New York, NY: Grosset & Dunlap, 2025.

Jackson, Tom. *The Small and Mighty Book of the Human Body*. London, UK: OH!, an imprint of Welbeck Children's Limited, 2023.

WEBSITES

How the Body Works
https://kidshealth.org/en/kids/center/htbw-main-page.html
Find out more about other body processes here.

What's Puke?
https://kidshealth.org/en/kids/puke.html
Read more about vomit here.

Publisher's note to educators and parents: Our editors have carefully reviewed these websites to ensure that they are suitable for students. Many websites change frequently, however, and we cannot guarantee that a site's future contents will continue to meet our high standards of quality and educational value. Be advised that students should be closely supervised whenever they access the internet.

INDEX